MOTIVATION MATTERS

UNLOCKING YOUR INNER DRIVE

AND ACHIEVING SUCCESS

EMMANUEL RILEY

Motivation Matters

Unlocking your Inner Drive

and Achieving Success

Fitness at Your Doorstep Volume 3

Copyright © 2023 by Emmanuel Riley

Other Titles by Emmanuel Riley

Fitness at Your Doorstep, Volume 1: Beginners Guide to Fitness

Fitness at Your Doorstep, Volume 2: Transformational Dietary Guide to Fitness

An Awareness Workbook: How Well Do You Know About Your Health and Fitness? (also available in Spanish)

Get in touch with Emmanuel Riley to request a copy: *teambeyondfitness@gmail.com*

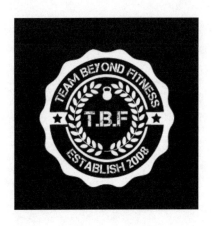

INTRODUCTION

Coach Manny is a fitness expert and wellness advocate who has dedicated his life to helping others achieve their health and fitness goals. With over a decade of experience in the fitness industry, Coach Manny has developed a reputation as a knowledgeable and passionate coach who truly cares about his clients. But Coach Manny's journey to becoming a fitness coach wasn't easy. He faced his own health challenges and setbacks, including open-heart surgery, which forced him to re-evaluate his life and his priorities. Through these experiences, he discovered a passion for fitness and wellness that he knew he had to share with others.

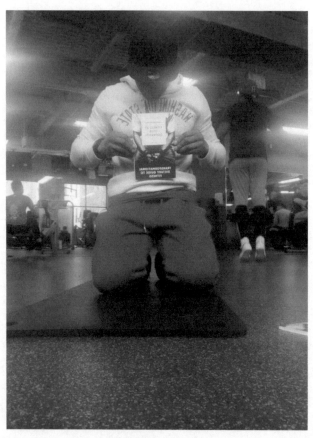

Since then, Coach Manny has been working tirelessly to help people get fit and healthy, no matter their age, fitness level, or circumstances. He's developed innovative fitness programs and written books on fitness and nutrition, all designed to help people achieve their goals and live their best lives.

But what sets Coach Manny apart isn't just his expertise and substantial knowledge. It's his tireless passion for his work and his deep sense of empathy and compassion for his clients. He understands that fitness isn't just about physical health; it's about mental and emotional well-being as well. Through his work, Coach Manny has touched countless lives and inspired people to make positive changes in their lives. He's a true leader in the fitness industry, and his dedication to his clients and his craft is an inspiration to us all.

Manny's perseverance in the face of his heart surgery is truly inspiring. Rather than procrastinating or giving up, he faced his challenges head-on with a determined and open heart. Despite the difficulties he encountered along the way, Manny remained focused on his goal and never lost sight of what was important to him.

Through his unwavering perseverance, Manny was able to overcome the obstacles in his path and emerge stronger and more resilient than ever before. His experience serves as a powerful reminder that with hard work and determination, we can overcome even the most daunting challenges and achieve our goals.

Have you ever been inspired by someone who has faced a major setback yet refused to give up on their dreams?

Coach Manny is one such individual who has touched countless lives through his work in the fitness industry. He's a true leader who has dedicated himself to helping his clients make positive changes in their lives. By sharing his story, Manny hopes to inspire others to embrace the power of perseverance and never give up on their dreams – no matter how difficult the road ahead may seem.

Whether facing personal struggles or professional setbacks, Manny's example motivates us to find the strength to keep moving forward with determination and an open heart.

A key part of living a good life is living healthily. When it comes to living a healthy life, there are a few simple guidelines to follow. Manny prioritizes eating healthily and making nutritious choices. By adopting a healthy diet, we can all learn how to live healthier lives and improve our overall well-being. Along with healthy eating, incorporating regular exercise, such as a gym routine, can also contribute to a healthy lifestyle. It's important to find a routine that works for you and fits into your schedule.

Over the years, Coach Manny has touched countless lives through his work. His clients consistently speak of his unwavering dedication to their success and his unique ability to motivate them to make positive changes in their lives. His passion for fitness and health is contagious, and he has become a true leader in the industry.

Coach Manny has already written four books on fitness and health, each one packed with valuable insights and practical tips to help readers achieve their goals. Manny's previous books cover the best ways to incorporate exercise into your daily life as well as offering a comprehensive guide to transforming your health and well-being through what you eat. And now, he's releasing his fifth book, which promises to be his best yet.

In his latest book, Coach Manny shares his own personal journey, including the setbacks he's faced along the way and the strategies he's used to overcome fear and negativity, motivating himself to go higher and achieve more.

Whether you're a seasoned fitness enthusiast or just starting out on your journey, Coach Manny's new book is a must-read. With his guidance and support, you too can achieve your goals and live the healthy, vibrant life you've always dreamed of.

So, what are you waiting for? Get ready to be inspired and motivated like never before.

1. Early Beginnings

On October 25, 1974, a special baby boy named Emmanuel Riley was born into the world. He was the creative and spiritual seed of life for the Johnson and Riley family, and his birth felt like a shift in the universe. Even before he was born, his parents signaled their vibration to the Universe, Emmanuel was already being shaped by the world around him while he was in his mother's womb.

Emmanuel's mother was only 19 years old and living under the influence of life in the streets. She was searching for guidance and direction, but despite the challenges, she was intelligent and self-conscious. She believed that she was ready for the world, and Emmanuel's faith has always been strong. He believed that God had left some instructions for him in His plan before birth. Greatness was already within him, waiting to be fully developed. He was created as a productive being – transparent as the tree of life.

Emmanuel Remembers

I remember my grandmother teaching me the value of saving money and not placing too much importance on material possessions. Although it was easy to get the things I wanted, I didn't see the value in material objects. I recall letting my friends borrow my belongings, and if they broke them, it didn't matter much to me. I knew I could easily replace them, but I didn't see those items as valuable.

Even at a young age, I knew I was special and had a purpose, though I wasn't quite sure what it was yet. I had a different kind of glow about me, and I stood out from the rest. I had a great personality, good energy, and was always physically fit. Girls were drawn to me, and people, in general, seemed to gravitate toward me, even if it wasn't always for the best reasons.

As I grew, I began to understand that these experiences were all part of life's journey, and I believe that God made it that way for a reason. Through the ups and downs, I learned the importance of valuing myself and my worth beyond just my material possessions. I realized that my true worth comes from within and that my energy, personality, and character are what truly set me apart from others.

Looking back, I am grateful for the lessons my grandmother taught me about saving money and not being too attached to material things. It allowed me to see the bigger picture and focus on what really matters in life: my purpose, my relationships with others, and my inner worth.

The Power of Life: The Seed Within Us

As humans, we often experience things in the moment, without fully understanding what we are experiencing. Life comes without instructions, and we are often unaware of the depths of human behavior. Many people do not reveal their true consciousness. Our selves can often be a distraction from our true purpose. However, God has planted the seed of greatness within us, choosing certain individuals to carry out his plan during our time on Earth. As human beings, we have the power to dominate and take care of the things on this planet, including the Kingdom of Heaven, which is more real than Earth in a biblical context.

The vibrations of energy we sustain are more significant than we can imagine. We pick up on energies and vibes, and not all individuals operate on the same frequency. Some vibrations are low, while others are high. High-vibration people have a strong sense of urgency and desire more out of life without making excuses. Conversely, low-energy people should pay attention to their body language, as it can work against them. No one can break you or take away your purpose. Your future has always been a part of you, from the moment you were a seed of life being harvested. The manifestation around you is guiding us toward our destiny.

Everything in life is a season, and your past does not define your future. As Dr. Myles Monroe said, "You should not believe what people tell you about your life; you should be the only one making decisions about your life." Set high standards for yourself and lead by example.

Live each day as though it were your last because, one day, you will be called for a new assignment, and you must be ready. Living may be the hardest assignment in life – it is often said that death is easier. Being alive for only a short amount of time comes with pain, suffering, responsibilities, and many other life tasks. So, it is essential to appreciate your life and make the best of it. It is best to be a giver rather than a taker – a lesson learned through wisdom and experience.

2. My Mother, My Inspiration

My mother was a beautiful woman in her prime with long, curly, thick hair and skin with a caramel complexion. Standing about 5 feet tall, she was an alpha female with her femininity and sexuality. I recall my mother being at her best during the winter, wearing her stunning suede shoes. She was a small woman with multiple talents and multiple fur coats – one of my favorites was a superb brown and white rabbit coat. Elegance personified!

Despite everything going on in her life, my mother kept her head high with pride and determination. Looking back, I realize that the struggles we faced gave her strength and I did my best to open her eyes to new perspectives. As a young woman with limited information, my mother did her best to navigate the world. I believe she was as aware as she could be, but she needed support and positive influence to remind her of her own greatness.

I was a special seed planted and growing in her body with an incredible purpose. It was my time to be introduced to the world, and I know that my mother loved me with every fiber of her being.

As I reflect on my mother's life, I believe that she could have made better choices if she had more knowledge and information at her fingertips. But despite her limitations, she had her own way of guiding me as a young boy. I still remember those times with fondness. In fact, my mother's strength and determination continue to inspire me to this day.

Despite the challenges she faced, she always tried to do her best for our family. I feel honored to have her as my mother and grateful for the lessons she taught me. I imagine it must have been overwhelming at times, but she loved me with every ounce of her soul. Now, I believe that she just needed some moral support and positive influence to remind her how great she was.

A combination of people and circumstances helped to shape my young mother and so helped to shape me. I remember being a young, happy, and intelligent boy at heart. I feel grateful to have had her as my mother. I will always remember the lessons she taught me – both good and bad.

A Snapshot of My Life

Nanna was transitioning from a situation in which she lived with her alcoholic husband before Momma's pregnancy with her young son who was finding his way in this world.

I did not meet Nanna in this lifetime. We will meet on the other side when my assignment is over in this place called Earth. Could it be that I was feeling Momma's emotions when she was carrying me inside her?

The picture I created in my head of my Momma carrying me, the seed of life, in that nice warm place where everything should be quiet and peaceful. Every human life form has experienced the biological connection between mother and child with the process developing inside. I always heard inspiring stories about Nanna. I heard her beauty was something to talk about. Nanna's mother was a fox as well, Great Gamma Honey-Child, with her high cheekbones followed by confidence and pride.

The higher power created me at those times to keep Momma on track, but I didn't know at the time what

Momma was trying to figure out. Momma had seen certain things in her younger years and was emulating Nanna's lifestyle. Nanna was a woman of variety when it came to men. Momma grew up fast with Nanna missing out on her life, dying when she was just 9. So, Momma having her baby boy at 20 years old was an experience of a lifetime.

Fight Your Battles

As women of color living in the struggling society of poverty in late Harlem, my family was well-known and respected for their influence in the community. Momma taught me how to protect myself in many ways. One of the main principles was not fearing any men and standing up for myself. This gave me a sense of authority over myself. I remember her showing me how to defend myself. I was only a young boy and not very strong. Weak children wouldn't have survived at that time, as my mother often reminded me.

Momma showed me that fighting my battles was the only way, and she always had my back like a true mom should. In fact, Momma would have taken a motherf***er out for me or any of our family. She was nicknamed Crazy K for a reason, lol.

Momma did what she could to make me happy by allowing me to spend quality time with my father and his mother, who later became like a mother to me as I grew into a young man. Growing up with Momma was really complicated at times. I think she just didn't understand the gifts she possessed, and in fact, she may have been completely unaware they existed.

In the next chapter, I will turn to the challenges of parenting and give some advice based on my observations and experiences over the years.

3. Parenting

Parenting can be challenging at times, especially when faced with difficult circumstances. However, I trust that you are determined to be intentional and deliver the best possible care for your child. Remember to also take care of yourself and seek support when needed, as parenting is a team effort. As the saying goes, it takes a village!!

While there may not be a one-size-fits-all guidebook for parenting, there are many resources available to help you along the way. Consider reaching out to parenting groups or seeking advice from trusted family and friends. And remember, at the end of the day, the most important thing you can give your child is your love and attention.

Throughout my life, I have been fortunate to have the love and support of people who cared for me unconditionally. Their guidance and nurturing have taught me important principles of life that I now strive to pass on to my own child.

As a young father, I recognized that raising a child would be a work in progress. I would need to develop my skills and understanding through intentional effort and hard work. Although I did not have a guidebook to follow, I was committed to being present for my child and providing her with the love and care that she needed to thrive. Despite facing challenges and living in a sometimes hostile environment, I remained – and remain – determined to be the best father I could – and can – be.

So, I sought out resources and support from parenting groups and trusted family and friends, learning valuable lessons along the way. As I continue on my parenting journey, I am reminded that there is no one-size-fits-all approach to raising a child. However, I am confident that with love, intentionality, and a willingness to learn and grow, I can provide my child with the foundation she needs to succeed in life.

P.S. I love you.

It is my responsibility to provide my daughter with the love and support that she needs to thrive, but I also wanted to do more than that — I wanted to set an example for her and for others who might be struggling to find their way. Therefore, I started writing down my thoughts and experiences, sharing words of encouragement and inspiration with anyone who would listen. I didn't have all the answers, but I knew that by sharing my story and the lessons I had learned along the way, I could help others find their own motivation and purpose in life. The result is the book you are currently reading as well as the other guides I have put together over the years. I have no plans to stop writing so get ready for more!

Dimonae Arella Riley: Light of My Life

My daughter, Dimonae Arella Riley, was born in 1996. From the moment I laid eyes on her, I knew she was also destined for greatness. So, I was aware that, as her father, the information and the lessons I gave to her would be critical in shaping her future.

My daughter grew up to be a true businesswoman, and she's doing great for herself. Dimonae has always had a strong work ethic and a drive to succeed, and I couldn't be prouder of her. Some might say she's clearly a version of me, but she also has her own unique talents and strengths. Watching Dimonae grow and flourish has been one of the greatest joys of my life.

Now, as a grandfather to her three children, I see the impact that my own teachings and the teachings of my ancestors have had on the next generation. Children truly do develop based on the information we instill in them and the lessons we teach them. It's up to us as parents and grandparents to instill positive values and provide guidance that will help them grow into kind, successful, and responsible adults.

It takes a village: Ways to serve your family and friends during difficult times

Here are a few clear, actionable ways to care for your family and friends so you can better serve your community.

1. Prioritize communication

I make sure to stay in touch with my family and friends regularly, even if it is just a quick phone call or text message with a few emojis. This helps us all feel less isolated and more connected.

2. Offer support

I reach out to people who I know are struggling, offering to help in any way I can. This included running errands, dropping off groceries, or just being a listening ear.

3. Adapt my services

As a service provider, I adapted my services to the new reality of the COVID-19 pandemic. This meant offering virtual services, creating new offerings that were more pandemic-friendly, and finding creative ways to continue serving my clients, recognizing the new reality.

4. Maintain focus on values

I made sure to maintain a focus on what mattered most to me — my family, friends, and community. This helped me stay grounded and focused on what was truly important during this challenging time.

5. Looked for opportunities to give back

I looked for ways to give back to my community, whether it was through volunteering or donating to a local charity. This helped me feel like I was making a positive impact during a difficult time.

Overall, revamping my approach to serving my family and friends during the pandemic helped me stay connected, focused, and positive during a challenging time.

In the following chapter, I reflect on my journey to finding purpose as a writer, father, and fitness coach.

4. Journey to Find Purpose

As I reflect on my life and the lessons I've learned, I know that my experiences can go a long way in helping others. That's why I'm sharing my story and my insights with the world. I hope that by sharing my experiences, I can inspire others to embrace their own challenges and find the positive in every situation.

Through writing, I find that my own sense of purpose and motivation has grown even stronger. I am no longer just a young man trying to figure out what would be next for me — I am a father, a writer, and a mentor to those who need support and guidance.

And as I have watched my daughter grow and thrive, I know that I am on the right path. She has always been my greatest motivation, my reason for striving to be the best version of myself. Today, my daughter is a young woman making her own way in the world, and I couldn't be prouder of her. And while my journey as a father and writer is far from over, I know that I am on the right path.

5. Fitness and Motivation

Fitness is much more than just physical exercise or athletic performance. It is a holistic concept that encompasses physical, mental, emotional, and even spiritual health. When we engage in fitness activities, we are not just improving our physical strength, endurance, and flexibility, but we are also developing ourselves as individuals.

One of the key ways in which fitness fosters personal development and growth is through the cultivation of discipline and perseverance. Regular exercise requires commitment and dedication, and it teaches us to push through challenges and setbacks. This translates to other areas of our lives, such as our careers, relationships, and personal goals. When we learn to persevere through difficult workouts or training regimes, we develop a sense of resilience and determination that can help us overcome obstacles in all areas of our lives.

Another way in which fitness contributes to personal growth is by promoting self-awareness and self-confidence. Engaging in physical activities allows us to learn about our bodies and our capabilities, and it can help us identify areas in which we want to improve – physically and mentally.

Fitness has a strong positive impact on our mental and emotional well-being. As we see progress in our fitness goals, we also build a sense of self-efficacy and confidence in our abilities. This can help other aspects of our lives – both personal and professional – as we become more willing to take risks and pursue new challenges. Exercise has also been shown to reduce symptoms of anxiety and depression, and it can help us manage stress and improve our mood.

By making time for self-care and prioritizing our fitness goals, we are also sending a message to ourselves that we value our health and well-being. Fitness is a powerful tool for personal development and growth. Engaging in regular physical activity can cultivate discipline, perseverance, self-awareness, and self-confidence. We can also improve our mental and emotional well-being and develop a sense of self-worth and purpose. Whether we are training for a marathon, practicing yoga, or simply going for a walk, each fitness activity is an opportunity to grow and become the best version of ourselves.

In the next chapter, I look in more detail at the idea of self-care and self-worth – vital building blocks of being the greatest version of yourself.

6. Self-care and Self-Worth

As young men and women, it's essential to recognize your self-worth and understand the value you bring to the world. Living a purposeful life with confidence, self-esteem, and integrity is key to building your character and self-love.

One of the most important things you can do to achieve your goals is to care for yourself before trying to care for others. This doesn't mean being selfish, but rather prioritizing your needs and well-being. In doing so, you'll build the confidence and self-belief necessary to accomplish anything you set your mind to. It's vital to remember that there is greatness within each and every one of us. You are special and unique, and no one can take that away from you. With hard work, dedication, and a little bit of self-belief, you can achieve anything you set your mind to.

As a spiritual being created for reproduction, you have inherent value and worth. However, without self-esteem, life can be an even more challenging road. If you don't believe in yourself, you won't understand the unique value you bring to the world as a human being, and you may feel unworthy. Remember, you are capable of achieving greatness, but it starts with believing in yourself and recognizing your own value.

Take the time to care for yourself, build your confidence and self-esteem, and live a purposeful life with integrity.

7. Identifying Your Motivation

Motivation is the driving force that pushes us to achieve our goals and live our best lives. It's the spark that ignites our passions and keeps us going even when we face obstacles or setbacks. But how do we find motivation when we feel stuck or unmotivated? How do we bring out the best in ourselves and tap into our full potential?

The first step is to identify what motivates us. Is it a specific goal like running a marathon or starting a business? Or is it a broader sense of purpose, like helping others or making a positive impact on the world?

Once we know what motivates us, we can begin to set goals and create a plan of action. This plan should be specific, measurable, and achievable – with clear deadlines and milestones along the way. It can also be helpful to break our goals down into smaller, more manageable steps. This not only makes them feel less daunting but also gives us a sense of progress and accomplishment as we check off each milestone.

Another key factor in finding motivation is our mindset. We must believe in ourselves and our ability to achieve our goals. We must be willing to take risks, make mistakes, and learn from them.

It's also important to surround ourselves with positive influences, like supportive friends and mentors who encourage us to reach our full potential. Their words of encouragement and wisdom can help us stay motivated and focused on our goals.

At the same time, we must also take care of ourselves, both physically and mentally. This means getting enough sleep, eating well, and exercising regularly, as well as practicing self-care activities like meditation or journaling. When we prioritize our well-being and surround ourselves with positive influences, we create an environment that fosters motivation and growth. We become more resilient in the face of challenges, more focused on our goals, and more confident in our ability to achieve them.

Overall, motivation is the key to unlocking our full potential and living our best lives. By identifying what motivates us, setting specific goals, and creating a plan of action, we can bring out the best in ourselves and achieve great things. By cultivating a positive mindset, surrounding ourselves with positive influences, and taking care of ourselves both physically and mentally, we can create a positive environment that fosters motivation and growth. So, let's tap into our inner drive, set our sights on our goals, and get motivated to achieve our dreams!

So, to anyone who may be struggling to find their own motivation or purpose in life, I would offer this advice: start by looking within yourself. Identify what drives you, what makes you feel alive and passionate. Then, set specific goals and create a plan of action to achieve them. Write down your thoughts and experiences and share them with others. And most importantly, never give up on yourself or your dreams. With hard work, determination, and a little bit of motivation, anything is possible.

Now, I turn to the vital notion of serving the community, particularly seniors, as well as give some tips on how you can help your loved ones even amid chaos and the challenges of our world today.

8. Serving the Community

For Seniors

I have been dedicated to working with senior citizens for over three years, creating fitness programs tailored specifically for seniors and producing content to help them stay healthy and active. Recently, I released a workbook, the culmination of hard work and dedication. I hope it helps many seniors stay fit and healthy for plenty of years to come.

I have always admired senior citizens, as they are the true pillars of my community – the keepers of its culture and traditions. So, when I started working with seniors three years ago, I knew that I had found my calling.

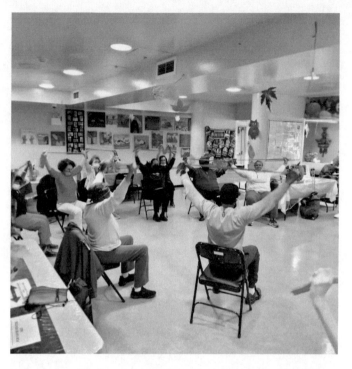

As I spent more time with seniors, I began to understand and appreciate their wisdom, integrity, and experience on a deeper level. I realized that they had so much to offer and that their contributions to the community were profoundly invaluable. I listened to their stories, learned from their experiences, and incorporated their ideas into my fitness programs.

Knowing that they are the ones who built the community means I realize that it is my responsibility to honor and preserve their legacy.

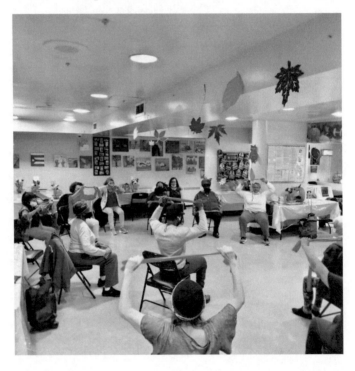

Through my work, I aim to empower senior citizens to live their lives to the fullest. I want them to be healthy, active, and engaged in the community. I believe that by doing so, they will continue to be an integral part of the community, inspiring future generations to carry on their legacy. I am determined to show them just how much they mean to the community. In essence, my work is a testament to my love for senior citizens and my belief in the power of community and culture.

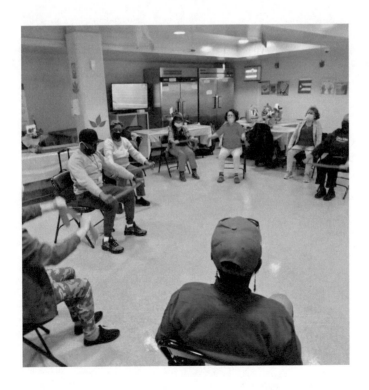

The next chapter turns to the event that changed my life and how I reinvented myself to become my current incarnation.

9. Reinventing Myself

Four years ago, I faced a life-threatening situation and had to undergo open-heart surgery. This was not only a physical ailment but also a significant emotional and financial setback. Shortly after my surgery, I lost my job, and I was left with nothing but my faith in a higher power to get me through. Despite this extremely difficult situation, I refused to give up. Taking accountability and responsibility for my situation, I decided to reinvent myself.

I realized my deep passion for fitness and wanted to help others achieve their goals. With this newfound sense of purpose, I wrote my first book, *Beginner's Guide to Fitness: Fitness at Your Doorstep*. This book is the culmination of my many years of experience and knowledge. It is designed to help people get fit and healthy from the comfort of their own homes. Through writing, I was not only able to share my story but also inspire others to take control of their lives. I knew that my life-threatening illness had actually saved my life; fundamentally, it was a test of my inner strength and resilience.

My story is a testament to the power of faith, perseverance, and self-belief. It demonstrates that even in the face of adversity, it's possible to turn things around and reinvent yourself. So, my books are designed as guides for anyone who wants to take control of their health and fitness and start living their best life.

In the end, my journey is a reminder that life is full of challenges, but it's also full of opportunities. It's up to us to embrace those opportunities, take responsibility for our lives, and create the future we want.

In addition to my other books, given the thriving Spanish-speaking community in the U.S. and globally, I wanted to create an accessible fitness workbook that was available in both English and Spanish. In doing so, I am committed to promoting cultural diversity and accessibility, making my work available for a wider audience, and contributing to the cultural knowledge and understanding of those who speak both languages. This dedication to inclusivity and desire to share my knowledge and insights with others, regardless of their background or language, I hope, is a reflection of my values and impact. My goal is that my work serves as a model for others who seek to make a positive impact on the world and promote cultural diversity.

10. Turning Challenges into Opportunities

As you have probably already realized from reading this book, I am passionate about making a positive impact in the world. I believe that we all have the power to make a difference and that we should use our time, influence, knowledge, and empathy to help others. I was inspired to pursue this path by my mother, who raised me as her only son and instilled in me a strong sense of responsibility to help those around me.

In my quest to make a difference, I have faced many challenges and fears. But I have learned to embrace these challenges and use them as motivation to keep pushing forward. I believe that men and women alike have a responsibility to motivate each other and work together to create a better world for our children and future generations.

I recognize that there are many systemic issues that have plagued our society for centuries, including colonialism, capitalism, and inequality. But I believe that it is time for us to take back what is rightfully ours and fight for a better future. By leveraging our collective knowledge, skills, and resources, we can work to create a new world order that prioritizes the well-being of all people and the planet.

I am committed to using my knowledge, intellectual and spiritual care, empathy, and influence to make a positive impact in the world. Whether through community service, activism, or other means, I am dedicated to making the world a better place for all.

The COVID-19 pandemic brought about a lot of changes in the world, including the way people run their businesses. Despite the economic downturn, many people from diverse backgrounds, including people of color, saw an opportunity to create and grow their own businesses to survive the pandemic.

One such person was a quick-thinking Black man who saw the potential for success during a time when the world seemed to be at a standstill. He recognized the urgency and need for revenue in the economic system and acted on it with determination and creativity… In fact, he wrote this book!!

It's clear that during the height of the pandemic, the hand of divine intervention was present. We needed a shake-up in the world, and this was it. We just had to be obedient and submit to God's will. Obedience is a value that is not only desired but required by God. Success can only be achieved through obedience to the Will of God: "If you are willing and obedient, you will eat the best from the land; but if you resist and rebel, you will be devoured by the sword" (Isaiah 1:18-20). In John 14:23, His Son Jesus says, "If anyone loves Me, he will obey My teaching." And in Proverbs 13:13, we hear, "He who scorns instruction will pay for it, but he who respects a command is rewarded." These are just three biblical extracts, but the importance of obedience is reinforced throughout the text. Submit to the Lord's Will and the world will open itself to you.

Although it was a little scary at first, with so much uncertainty and confusion, I persevered and was able to make a substantial amount of money during this time of crisis. My business gains were impressive, and I was able to revamp my business strategy to adapt to the changing times.

Part of my success can be attributed to prioritizing precision in my professional (and personal) life. Being accurate and exact in your life is the secret to success in business, exercise, and beyond. This can mean anything from great form when doing pull-ups to making sure you're on time for meetings and appointments. People appreciate precision, even if they don't actively recognize it.

In conclusion, opportunities can arise during times of great crisis. My story is one of resilience, creativity, and determination and will hopefully serve as inspiration to those who have faced and continue to face similar challenges. Despite difficulties, as my own experience shows, it's possible to succeed and thrive in the face of adversity.

Some Final Thoughts

This book is about the power of self-awareness and how it can be harnessed to drive motivation and success in the economic system we live in. Through my personal experiences, I have discovered that being in touch with one's own inspirations and motivations is crucial to achieving success in all areas of life.

I stress the importance of exercise, not just for physical health but for overall well-being. I believe that access to exercise should be a priority for everyone and that it should be integrated into daily routines and healthcare. By making exercise a part of our social lives and environment, we can create a healthier, more active lifestyle.

But I don't stop at promoting exercise — I also emphasize the role of self-awareness in being successful. By understanding our own motivations and values, we can make better decisions and take actions that align with our goals. This, in turn, can lead to greater success in our careers and personal lives.

In this book, and elsewhere in my work, I have provided practical strategies for developing self-awareness and setting realistic goals. By breaking down the process into manageable steps, I hope readers can begin to take control of their own lives and achieve the success they desire.

Overall, this book is a call to action for readers to embrace tools like self-awareness and exercise to succeed in all areas of their lives. It's a powerful reminder that by being in touch with ourselves, we can unlock our full potential and achieve our dreams.

As a Black man, I know first-hand the obstacles that come with living in a society that has historically undervalued and disrespected people of color. Despite these challenges, we have always shown resilience and a willingness to work harder and smarter to achieve our goals.

When it comes to personal development, there is no one-size-fits-all system that will work for everyone. However, there are certain strategies that can be helpful in creating a successful healthcare approach. For example, establishing a support group can provide a sense of community and accountability, making it easier to stay motivated and on track.

Communication and support are also key components of an effective healthcare strategy. It's important to have a clear plan in place for how to communicate with healthcare providers, family members, and other support systems. This can involve setting up regular check-ins, using technology to stay connected, and having a backup plan in case of emergencies.

Finally, creating a system for payment and funding is essential for ensuring that healthcare is accessible to all. This can involve researching different insurance options, setting up a payment plan, or seeking out financial assistance programs.

In conclusion, personal development is a journey that requires dedication, hard work, and a willingness to seek out support when needed. By creating a healthcare plan that prioritizes community, communication, and accessibility, you can take control of your health and well-being and achieve your goals.

Postscript: How to Make Passive Income from Books

I wanted to share with you how I turned my books into a passive income stream from 2019 onwards. It wasn't easy, but it was definitely worth the effort.

First, I wrote and published my books. This was a lot of work, but I knew that if I could create something valuable and interesting, it could potentially generate income for me in the future.

Next, I had to market my books. I used social media, email marketing, and advertising to get the word out about my books and to attract potential readers. It took some time, but eventually, my books started to sell.

At first, I was actively promoting my books to generate sales and income. But over time, as my books gained popularity and began to sell consistently, they started to generate passive income. This meant that I no longer had to actively promote my books to generate sales and income – they were selling on their own.

Now, my books are a reliable source of passive income for me. I don't have to actively work on them, but I still earn money from their sales. This has allowed me to focus on other projects and activities, while still earning some income.

If you're interested in creating a passive income stream from something you've created, it's definitely possible. It will require some effort and upfront investment, but if you can create something valuable and attract an audience, you can potentially turn it into a reliable source of passive income.

It's wonderful that you have a desire to make a positive impact on society and inspire others. I assume that's the case as you're reading this book!! Expressing gratitude for the blessings in our lives is a great way to start each day with a positive mindset.

It's also admirable that you've learned from your mistakes and are using your gift to help others. Writing can be a powerful tool for self-reflection and sharing our experiences with others. I wish you the best of luck in your endeavors.

Afterword

Has life changed for people in the past 20 years? It's difficult to make a blanket statement as everyone's experiences are unique. However, we do know that humans are constantly evolving and adapting to new challenges and opportunities. And while some may experience negative changes, it's important to remember that we have the power to shape our own futures and make positive changes in our lives and communities. This book is about the impact and development of one man: Emmanuel Riley.

Manny's upbringing was a unique experience that shaped him into the person he is today. Unlike many others, Manny had to develop courage, self-esteem, character, and self-confidence at a young age. He faced challenges that required him to rely on his inner strength and resilience to overcome them.

Through it all, Manny's mother was his anchor. She played a crucial role in planting the seeds of these important qualities in him and nurturing them as they began to grow. Manny's mother was a constant source of encouragement and support, providing him with the love and guidance he needed to thrive.

As time went on, Manny's efforts began to bear fruit. He built a strong foundation filled with the values and principles that he had been taught. He became a person of integrity, with a deep sense of self-awareness and confidence radiating from within. He was equipped with the tools he needed to face life's challenges head-on, and he did so with grace and determination.

Manny's story is a testament to the power of a strong foundation and the importance of having someone in your corner to help you along the way. His journey is an inspiration to us all, reminding us that with hard work, perseverance, and a little bit of help from those we love, we can achieve anything we set our mind to.

Acknowledgments

I am deeply grateful to the individuals who have supported and encouraged me throughout this journey of writing this book. Their unwavering belief in me has been a constant source of inspiration and motivation.

I would especially like to thank my family and friends for their love, patience, and understanding. I am also indebted to my editor for their invaluable guidance and expertise, which has helped me to shape and refine my ideas.

Finally, I would like to express my deepest appreciation to the readers for their interest and support. This book would not have been possible without you. Thank you.

Learn more with *Fitness at Your Doorstep* by Emmanuel Riley

Fitness at Your Doorstep, Volume 1: Beginners Guide to Fitness

Fitness at Your Doorstep, Volume 2: Transformational Dietary Guide to Fitness

An Awareness Workbook: How Well Do You Know About Your Health and Fitness? (also available in Spanish)

Bio

Emmanuel Riley is a renowned fitness instructor from Harlem who has been dedicated to helping his community through fitness for over 12 years. He is particularly proud of his work with senior citizens over the past four years, helping them to stay active and healthy.

Emmanuel's passion for fitness serves as his motivation to create his own lane in the industry. He has authored five published books and workbooks, which showcase his expertise in the field.

Emmanuel is a firm believer in the importance of family. Emmanuel's grandchildren are the most valued part of his life. He loves spending time with them and cherishes every moment. Beyond his family, he is committed to making a positive impact on the world through his work.

To learn more about fitness and be guided on your health journey, get in touch via Instagram or email for personalized advice.

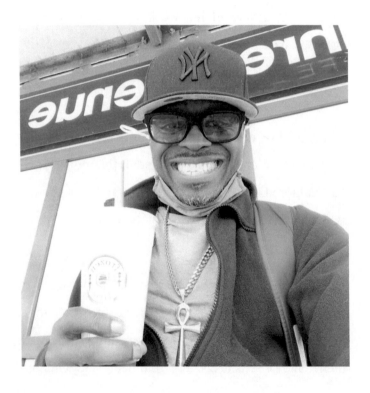

Be on the lookout for more books and workbooks!

Emmanuel Riley

Instagram: *@mannyblack123*

Email: *teambeyondfitness@gmail.com*

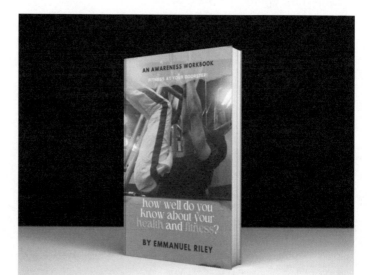

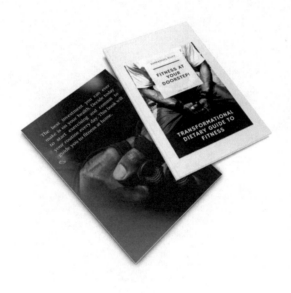

Made in the USA
Columbia, SC
06 May 2024

35343168R00041